THE ESSENTIAL KETO DIET BOOK FOR BEGINNERS

Lose Weight with Easy and Tasty Recipes incl. 30 Days Weight Loss Challenge

Olivia C. Robinson

ISBN- 9798661292070

TABLE OF CONTENTS

The Essential Keto Diet Book For Beginners

What is Keto?

Keto finds its foundation from LCHF (Low Carb High Fat).

The main principle you should stick to is a low carbohydrate level in your everyday ration.

Why the carbohydrates are not something that you need?

Following the habitual nutrition systems, your body works on glucose obtained from carbohydrates and proteins.

In the digestive tract of humans and animals, the carbohydrates are hydrolyzed and converted into glucose that is absorbed by the organism.

From the school biology and anatomy course, we know that glucose is fuel, that is, our energy. All the fibers of our body: brain, heart, lungs, muscles, kidneys - need it.

In order to deliver the glucose to consumers the pancreatic starts working. It produces insulin that transports the glucose in each cell.

Having delivered the glucose in cells, insulin begins to reduce because its permanently high level is not envisaged by nature. After 1-2 hours you will feel a pang of hunger and your hand will reach for a snack. This condition is called «insulin swings»

In keto diet not glucose provides us with a vital activity but ketones. While working on ketones your insulin is not jumping but stays stable because unlike carbohydrates, fats are broken down very slowly releasing ketones, which serve as energy.

Ketones are an alternative energy source that our body uses more effectively than glucose fuel.

Ketosis is the state of metabolism when fat coming with food is recycled by the liver in ketones.

To reach the ketos condition it is not enough to lower the carbohydrate intake as it is on a low carbohydrate level. It is necessary to adhere to certain proportions and correlations between proteins, fats and carbohydrates.

The ketos formula is the following:

- 20% - proteins
- 75% - fats
- 5% - carbohydrates

By only following these proportions for some time, your body will be able to produce ketones and get into ketos.

After all, keto is not only about the numbers on the scales, grams in plates, not about replacing sugar with stevia, but a banana with raspberries!

Keto is about well-being.

Adhering to keto nutrition you will reach a desirable weight without raping yourself, without stress and permanent hunger sense. You notice results and you want to move ahead because it acts like a motivation, you don't want to rest on its laurels.

Keto is about qualitative and natural products.

Following this diet, the preference should be given to unprocessed, qualitative, wholesome products, that give energy and satisfaction from delicious organic food.

Keto is about the normal hormonal background.

In addition to insulin, on keto or low carb diets improvements are also being noted in other body systems. Leptin is normalized - the hormone of satiety, and testosterone, that is responsible for sexual desire.

Types of Keto diet

1) **Standard diet.** This diet consists of low content of carbohydrates and proteins and high content of fats. Usually this diet contains 75% fat, 20% protein, and only 5 % of carbohydrates.

2) **Cyclic diet:** This diet includes periods high in carbohydrates, such as 5 ketogenic days, followed by 2 days high in carbohydrates.

3) **Target diet:** This diet allows adding carbohydrates in your ration during the workout.

4) **High-protein diet:** This diet is similar to the ketogenic diet but contains more proteins. The proportion frequently comprises 60% fat, 35% protein and 5% carbohydrates.

Nevertheless, only standard and high protein keto diets have been studied thoroughly.

Cyclic or target keto diets are more advanced methods and are mainly used by bodybuilders or athletes.

The effectivity of the keto diet

Many kinds of studies have shown that the keto diet is extremely effective and helpful for the human organism. Because of its high efficiency in fighting fat deposits, it has become famous among both celebrities and ordinary people. On average, you can lose 3-6 pounds depending on how much excess fat you have at the initial level.

Such rapid weight loss has become possible as the body is reconstructed to get energy from fats and it starts consuming the reserves of subcutaneous fat in conditions of calorie deficiency in the diet.

Basic principles and rules

Steps or keto principles are extremely easy to take.

1) Cut down on carbohydrates

2) Increase the consumption of healthy fats that will help to create satiety sense

3) Without glucose, your body will constrainedly burn fat and produce ketones

4) As soon as the level of ketones in the blood increases to a certain level, you will reach ketosis.

5) This condition leads to a consistent, fairly quick weight loss until your body reaches a healthy and stable weight.

Entering the Keto diet

The classic ketogenic diet - is a purely low-carb diet that was originally developed in the 1920s for epilepsy patients by researchers at the Johns Hopkins Medical Center. The researchers discovered that starvation – refusal from consuming all foods for a short period, including carbohydrates - helped to reduce the number of seizures suffered by patients, in addition to other beneficial effects - body fat reduced, blood sugar level, cholesterol level, hunger sense is normalized.

Unfortunately, prolonged starvation is an unacceptable option for an extended period. Thereby, this keto-diet was designed to mimic the same beneficial effects of fasting. It works by «tricking» the body, causing it to think that it is fasting (thus benefiting from starvation) by removing glucose and carbohydrate foods from the diet. Today, the standard keto diet has several different names, including "low carbohydrate" or "fatty".

The basis of the classic keto diet is a strict restriction on the consumption of all or most foods with sugar and starch (carbohydrates). These products decay into sugar (glucose) in our blood, but if the level becomes too high then extra calories are stored in the form of fat that causes an undesirable weight gain. However, when the glucose level is decreased due to its low carbohydrate intake, the organism starts to burn fat and produce ketones that can be measured.

When you follow a keto diet, your body burns fat to obtain the energy, not carbohydrates! Many people lose weight and extra fat rapidly when consuming a big amount of fat and sufficient calories every day. One more advantage of keto-diet is that there is no need in counting calories, feeling hungry or trying to burn calories for several hours by tantalizing yourself with an intensive and exhausting workout.

It resembles the Atkins diet that also boosts fat-burning organism ability on account by consuming low carbohydrate products as well as getting rid of high carbohydrate and sugar foods. Having cut the carbohydrate foods out of your diet, you induce your organism to burn fat with a view to obtaining energy. The main difference between classic keto and the Atkins diet is that in the first case, healthy fats, less protein, and additional studies confirming the effectiveness of the keto diet are emphasized.

What is ketosis?

Ketosis is the result of compliance with a standard keto diet that is why it is called sometimes ketose diet. This happens when the consumption of carbohydrate products is rapidly reduced (like cereals, sugar, and fruits) that forces the organism to look for an additional energy source - fat. Such condition can also be reached after several days of complete fasting but It cannot be sustained after several days of starvation. (This is why some keto diets combine periodic fasting with a keto diet for a greater weight loss effect.)

Although notorious fat in your nutrition (particularly saturated fat) causes the fear of weight gain and heart disease, it is also the second preferred energy source for your organism when carbohydrates are unavailable.

In the absence of glucose, that is always used by cells as an additional energy source, the human body starts to burn fat and due to this produces ketone bodies. Once the level of ketones in the blood rises to a certain point, you go into a state of ketosis - which usually leads to a quick and permanent weight loss until you reach a healthy, stable body weight.

As a result of a complex biochemical process, you reach a state of fat burning when the liver breaks down fat into fatty acids and glycerin, through a process called beta-oxidation. There exist three major types of ketone bodies, which are water-soluble molecules produced in the liver: acetoacetate, beta-hydroxybutyrate and acetone.

Then the organism decomposes these fatty acids into energy-rich substances called ketones, which circulate in the blood. Fatty acid molecules are broken down by a process called ketogenesis, and a specific ketone substance called acetoacetate is formed, which supplies the body with energy.

So, what are the advantages of the Keto diet?

1. Satiety sense and release from constant thoughts about food.

Ketones are long energy so hunger sense doesn't bother you. There are no obsessive thoughts about food, you don't look at the clock waiting for lunch, you don't carry packed lunches and snacks along with you. You are free!

2. Physical health improvement

You eat whole, high-quality foods with minimal industrial processing. And food trash, like white flour, sugar, and other food packed with carbohydrates you simply are not interested in. You already know how this "works" against you and what it does with your body.

3. Psycho-emotional condition

Angry because you are hungry it is not about Keto!

4. Cognitive indicators enhancement- memory, attention, concentration.

On account of the absence of products that cause inflammatory processes (surplus of omega 3 fatty acids (seeds oils, gluten, sugar) in our nutrition, then our brain is cleansed and everything goes well.

5. A comfortable weight loss

When you switched from glucose to ketone way to get the energy, you start burning your fat stocks easily even if the energy from food is finished already. In addition, on the account of long satiety sense you easily create a comfortable calorie deficiency, the deficiency that won't be reflected on your general wellbeing and perfectly will work for the overall result.

6. Long-term result

Keto is not a diet and a short-term measure to fit your dress for a corporate party. Keto is a lifestyle. It is your ration planning, quality care products and sleep patterns. This is a directed and conscious work, the result which pleases you for a long time.

7. Decreased risk of cardiovascular diseases

A keto diet can reduce the risk of heart disease markers, including high cholesterol and triglycerides. Moreover, it can reduce the risk factors of cardiovascular diseases, especially for those people who are obese.

For example, studies have shown that following a ketogenic diet for 24 weeks resulted in lower levels of triglycerides, LDL cholesterol (bad cholesterol) and blood glucose in a significant percentage of patients, while increasing HDL (good) cholesterol levels.

8. Cancer protection

Some studies have shown that keto-diets can kill cancer cells by starvation. Low nutrient anti-inflammatory foods can nourish cancer cells causing them to reproduce. So, what is the connection between high consumption of sugar and cancer? Ordinary cells in our body can use fat to produce energy, but research has shown that cancer cells cannot metabolize the use of fat instead of glucose.

There are several medical studies, for example, two conducted by the Department of Radiation Oncology at Holden University of Cancer show that the ketogenic diet is an effective treatment for cancer and other serious health problems.

Consequently, the keto diet that rules out sugar consumption and other carbohydrates can be effective in fight with cancer or its prevention. It is not a coincidence that some of the best products in the fight against cancer are on the keto diet list.

9. Increases lifespan

There is evidence that a low-carb, high-fat diet (like a keto diet) prolongs the life and slows the senility process down. A keto diet also appears to help induce autophagy, which helps to eliminate damaged cells from the body, including aging cells that do not function but remain in tissues and organs.

Everything written of course looks great, but the keto diet has also disadvantages and contraindications that everyone who starts dieting should be aware of!

1. Like any other nutrition diet system, the Keto diet cannot suit you personally.

If you feel uncomfortable then it is not your nutrition style. (but don't confuse this condition with the lack of a desirable result after 3 days of following this diet or laziness to cooking)

2. Keto is not a good idea for children, pregnant women and breastfeeding mothers.

Liberal low-carb nutrition- yes. Strict keto diet-no!

3. Keto-flu.

Muscular weakness, fatigue, irritability and headache- is the result of the organism's adaptation to new conditions. Don't worry - it will leave you after a while.

Drink plenty of water, don't be afraid of consuming salt, light physical activity, and additional minerals intake will help you relieve your health condition.

4. Keto-rash.

Don't worry, not all people can experience this but more likely that overweight people will face this problem. Because subcutaneous fat had been accumulating decay products and other toxins in itself for years or even decades.

Fat is consumed, toxins are released, sometimes it is manifested in the form of a rash. It is not a dangerous condition requiring special intervention, it passes over time.

5. Acetone smell for the first time.

Acetone is a final product of ketones breakdown. Basically, it is excreted with urine, respiration and sweat. The smell becomes pungent and persistent, causing inconvenience for its owner with a lack of body fluids.

With the increase of the consumed amount of fluid and minerals, the use of chewing gum perfectly copes with this problem.

6. Defecation problems during the adaptation period

Reducing carbohydrate intake as a source of fiber, e.g. oatmeal, bran, whole grains, fruits, affects intestinal motility. Water, minerals, plus a little time to adapt and everything will be OK.

Keto beginners' mistakes

1. Speeding up the process.

Keto or low-carb diets don't show quick results. Be calm, give your organism to adapt and you will see how grateful it will be. You shouldn't immediately take on the most stringent option of the low carbohydrate nutrition. Try to keep track of your reactions and your body itself will choose a comfortable pace for it.

2. Focusing on weight.

If you need any numbers- you should better guide the volumes, keep the record of your body changes relying on your clothes. The most optimal variant is to be weighed once a week, or better - in two weeks.

Weight loss will not happen at the same rate constantly. If in the first month you lost 10 pounds, this absolutely doesn't guarantee the same progress in the following one.

3. Comparing yourself and your results with others'

Everybody is different and has different metabolism speed, another way of life, and the end of the day different weight.

Exhale, relax and enjoy the process. Compare new yourself to past yourself by clothes, by well-being, but only with yourself!

4. Not having a focus on wellbeing.

You should listen to yourself and get a kick out of everything you do or eat. Your comfortable organism response should take precedence.

5. Insufficient or poor-quality sleep.

Sleep is a very important component of a low-carb diet.

6. The absence of the nutrition plan in the first weeks

If you haven't mastered this technique and don't have a trained eye then you must draw up a detailed menu. This will allow you to significantly reduce the time for cooking, and save a decent amount of money when doing shopping sprees, and certainly will protect you from disruption.

7. The lack of water

To help the body flush out toxins that start to exude from accumulated fat over the years - you need to increase the consumption of drinking water. So, to make the adaptation process of the digestive tract go more easily you need to drink more water.

8. Neglect of minerals and vitamins.

Keto and low-carb nutrition systems differ from your usual everyday nutrition. Therefore, your body needs support. From the first days of the diet, you should pay special attention to additional minerals intake.

9. The protein surplus

You should strictly follow keto proportions - 20% protein from the total calorie content. Excess protein triggers glucose synthesis and you exit ketosis. The excess of protein, in conditions of restriction of carbohydrates, is fraught with kidney stress.

10. Lack of fat

If you consume not enough fat – you have no sufficient energy! Proportions are extremely important. If you have a low-carb diet, then lack of fat will affect your feeling of satiety

11. Wrong products

Keto is not just fatty fat. It's right fat! Sausages, mayonnaise from the store are not the best decision! These are quality, healthy products, with minimal industrial processing: whole meat, quality oil (unrefined and seedless), the right vegetables, the lack of gluten and cereals.

11. Snacks

Snacks during keto diet are your past habits. If your ration made up correctly then there is no need for snacks.

The most asked beginners' questions about the keto and low-carb diets

What about heart stroke and cholesterol level?

Low carb diet with a high level of healthy fats leads to the improvement of lipid profile- the number of triglycerides is decreased and «good» cholesterol is increased. These indicators demonstrate a lower risk of heart diseases.

More attention should be paid to blood sugar level since carbohydrates play a certain role in heart diseases. As a rule, a high blood sugar level increases the likelihood that bad cholesterol will harm your blood vessels and heart.

What are the contraindications for keto and low-carb nutrition systems?

Strict Keto is not recommended for:

- pregnant and lactating, as well as children (except treatment of certain diseases under the supervision of doctors)
- people with high blood pressure (possibly under doctor's supervision)
- people with insulin-dependent diabetes (possibly only under medical supervision)

How often and how much to eat during keto diet?

Remember that you need to eat only when you are hungry. Someone is comfortable with 3 meals a day, and someone feels great if eating 1-2 times a day. The only thing to be guided by is hunger and saturation. Eat slowly and consciously.

Is the diet safe for kidneys?

Yes! Both keto and low-carb diets are safe for kidneys since they are associated with high fat consumption but not protein. In fact, a keto diet can even protect your kidneys, especially if you have diabetes.

Keto and alcohol?

You should be careful with alcohol during the weight loss phase. From the scientific point of view, there is a danger of extra fat accumulation but practically-alcohol decreases your control level increases the risk of eating more than you plan.

Also, give preference to clean and simple drinks, avoiding added sugar. For example, in cocktails but usually, keto and alcohol have no direct contraindication.

How much and how fast can I lose weight?

It is very individual and can vary from 0.5 to 2.5 kg per week. It depends on your metabolic rate, age and activity level, etc. Focus on volume, not weight.

Is Keto compatible with veganism or vegetarianism?

Everything depends on your everyday rules and food preferences. If you allow dairy products and eggs in your diet, then you will be able to get all the necessary nutrients, including enough fat while practicing keto or low-carb diet.

If you are a definite vegan – a ketogenic vegetarian diet is not a good variant for you. Thereby, vegans exclude all the animal products. They must rely on a combination of grains, legumes and seeds, to get all the necessary macronutrients. For this reason, Keto and a vegetarian diet work poorly together.

Is it allowed to eat fruits on a diet?

Fruits contain too many carbohydrates. One eaten apple is unlikely to throw you out of ketosis, but to suspend fat burning – easily. Berries are preferable to fruits.

How to quit keto diet correctly?

Many people who have tried ketogenic nutrition, make this nutrition system their lifestyle. If you want to use a keto diet only until you reach your goal, then getting out of it will not be difficult. Just gradually add more protein and carbohydrates to your diet.

Keto on a budget. Make it happen.

The most common ways to do the keto diet on a budget.

When you start thinking of keto diet the typical products that come up to your mind are salmon, turkey, shrimps, or tuna. Buying such foods can be quite expensive. Still, if you finally have made a decision to follow the keto diet and are sure that it is the right for you there exist some ways to do it on budget and not lose your T-shirt while being on this diet.

Here are 8 the most common ways to save money while doing the ketogenic diet:

1. Buy and cook in bulk.

Buying in bulk you get a great opportunity to do keto diet on a budget. When you find a great deal take advantage of it. Stock up by purchasing such items as seasonings, coconut flour and milk, pantry essentials by the case. Seafood and meat can put a serious dent in your grocery bill. So, if you come across meat on sale, buy more than you need and freeze for a rainy day. Also, purchase several bags of frozen vegetables and store them properly. Yes, fresh vegetables are tastier but frozen much more affordable. If you already buy the food in bulk so cook in bulk as well.

2. Freeze any leftovers.

If in one week you are cooking more than you can eat, just freeze what you don't use. Most people think that a deep freezer is a good investment moreover if you have the space available. It helps you to prepare and store those budget-friendly finds well in advance.

3. Always write down a shopping list in advance and stick to it.

If you have a ready written shopping list then there is no risk of buying something unnecessary. Without a precise list of what you plan to buy there is a 99% likelihood you will surely buy more than planned. Impulse purchases are a real thing. Always go on a shopping spree with a list and buy only you that you took down.

4. Look for Offers and Discounts

Always take advantage of deals and discounts when you shop at the grocery store. When meat nears its expiration date, stores often discount it by as much as 20%. If you prepare meals each day, this is a great opportunity for you to bump into high-quality, grass-fed meat at incredibly low prices.

BOGO (buy one, get one) deals are another popular grocery store promotion. In the food and butcher pages, look for BOGO offers, then scan the aisles for pantry staples-related offerings. That way, you can actually do keto on a budget, so get used to checking weekly flyers and ads in-store for good offers and coupons.

5. Shop online.

If you can't find deals locally, shopping online can significantly save money. Amazon has a number of low-priced deals concerning nuts, coconut flour, coconut oil or milk, almond flour, chia or flax seeds or seasonings.

6. Use FoodSaver

A FoodSaver is a vacuum for sealing and extracting air from the plastic bags. You can freeze meals and avoid freezer burning by using a FoodSaver. A Bonus Added? It frees up space in the freezer that you will need to buy and cook over bulk.

7. Notice if your grocery bill goes to beverages not food.

If you are whining about your food bill and spend $7 every single day on a latte or coffee here is a frustrating realization- latte is not even food. And every time you visit the store you are buying a $20 bottle of wine (or worse, charging a $50 bar tab every Thursday at a happy hour), those line items add up.

Go cold turkey with the expensive drinks and alcohol and give the preference to water. If you need caffeine, make homemade coffee or tea and carry it in a mug. Regarding alcohol, you should probably cut back altogether — it's full of sugar anyway.

8. Opt for Eggs and get healthy fat for free

Eggs are one of the most economically advantageous products and are completely keto-friendly. One big egg consists of 4,8 fat, 0,4 carbohydrates, and 6,3 protein.

What to eat during keto diet?

Keto and low-carb ration is diversified, balanced (with a well-prepared nutrition plan), and very delicious.

Next, you will be acquainted with products that are allowed and forbidden during keto diet

Allowed	Allowed in moderation	Forbidden
Oils: • butter • ghee • olive oil • coconut oil • peanut butter	Milk Cottage cheese	Meat intermediate goods: • sausages • delicacies
Meat: • beef • pork • mutton • turkey • venison	Industrial Grown Chicken	**Seed oils:** • sunflower • corn • vegetable • rapeseed • soy

Allowed	Allowed in moderation	Forbidden
Fish and seafood: • Alaska pollock • Cod • Mackerel • Plaice • Herring • Salmon • Squids	Legumes: • Chickpeas • Beans • Lentil	Mayonnaise • Ketchup • Margarine • Canned sauces
Dairy products: • Cream • Sour cream • Hard cheese	Carrot Beetroot Nuts	**Bakery goods:** • Macaroni • Potato • Rice • Porridges
Eggs	Low carbon ang gluten free products	• Sugar • Honey • Big amount of fruits
Vegetables: • All kinds of cabbage • Salad leaves • greenery	Fruits and berries(seasonal)	**Juices:** • Fresh • Sweet smoothies • Cocktails

1, 2, 3 let's get started!

If you have read before this chapter, then you are determined to change your food habits and become healthy and slim!

A journey of a thousand miles begins with one step.

1. The very first step is to revise your fridges, pantries and closets!

With no regret throw away:

- **Sunflower and all kinds of harmful oils**

- **All sources of gluten:** wheat flour, including "such healthy "whole grain, pasta, oatmeal, cooked breakfasts, cookies, crackers, sweet snacks, sweets, soy sauce

- **All types of starches:** potato, corn

- **Sugar** (white, brown, coconut and any other), honey. Everything that contains added sugar: sauces, ketchup, juices, syrups, chemical sweeteners

- **Cereals** are a source of carbohydrates and insulin surges. But if you can't imagine your life without buckwheat, you can leave it for the first time no more than once a week

- **All sweets:** ice cream, chocolate (even dark chocolate contains sugar), and jams

- **All convenient food:** processed cheese, sausages, cutlets, canned pastes

2. The second step - go to the store and give preference to seasonal, environmentally friendly local products.

- Olive, coconut, camelina butter and ghee

- Eggs, farm poultry, pork, beef, lamb, game

- High-quality fat cheeses (no inscriptions "cheese

- product")
- The fattest cream and rustic sour cream, a little greasy cottage cheese
- Cabbage, cauliflower, Brussels, Beijing, sauerkraut,
- Broccoli, celery, radish, avocado, herbs, leafy lettuce, zucchini, eggplant, mushrooms, etc.
- Berries. Frozen is no worse than fresh
- Pumpkin, flaxseed, sesame seeds. Walnuts, almonds, pecans, hazelnuts
- Coconut, almond, linseed flour. No rice flour doesn't contain gluten, but is too carbohydrate. It can be used in rare cases and limited quantities.
- Safe sweeteners erythritol, stevia, erythritol and stevia)

3. Constitute a menu for a week and stick to a nutrition plan!

By doing this, you will learn how to form the right food habits and adapt to a new ration. It will also save you from impulsive purchases and unjustified expenses.

In the first 2-4 weeks it is desirable to eat homemade food so that you can concentrate on the quality of dishes and their composition. After all, you know exactly what oil you fried cutlets in and that they don't contain bread and semolina, and you didn't add starch or sugar to the sauce.

Each meal of the day must consist of healthy fats and proteins. There are no restrictions concerning vegetables except for potato, corn, and carrot.

At the stage of weight loss, still keep the standards of the calorie content according to your plan or menu.

4. Move to 3-meals per day. Without snacks!

Breakfast at 8-10 am, lunch at 1-3 pm and dinner at 7pm but orientate on hunger sense.

If it is high time to have lunch but you are not hungry yet then you don't have to force yourself.

5. Focus on sleep quality and quantity

This point is critical because the production of the satiety hormone Leptin directly depends on the quality and quantity of Melatonin hormone that is produced during sleeping.

In other words, the less you sleep the more you eat on the following day.

6. Be consistent and flexible, not fanatically adamant.

Don't tantalize yourself and don't impose severe penalties for an accidentally eaten piece of pizza or cake.

The most important thing is to stop on time and come back on the right path. The longer you follow low-carb or keto nutrition, the easier your attitude to food and its selection becomes.

And of course, keep in mind the advantages of low-carb and keto

High-fat and low-carb diets help to get rid of cravings for certain foods (mainly

flour and sweet), avoid mental stagnation that occurs in the afternoon, increase mental activity and control hunger and calorie content.

A simple example of keto diet for a week

Monday

Breakfast: bacon, eggs and tomatoes
Lunch: chicken salad with olive oil and feta cheese
Dinner: salmon with asparagus cooked in butter.

Tuesday

Breakfast: omelet with egg, tomato, basil and goat cheese.
Lunch: almond milk, peanut butter, cocoa powder and milkshake with sweetener
Dinner: Meatballs, Cheddar Cheese and Vegetables.

Wednesday:

Breakfast: ketogenic milkshake
Lunch: shrimp salad with olive oil and avocado.
Dinner: pork chops with parmesan, broccoli and salad.

Thursday:

Breakfast: omelet with avocado, salsa, pepper, onions and spices
Lunch: A handful of nuts and celery with guacamole and salsa.
Dinner: chicken stuffed with pesto and cream cheese, along with vegetables.

Friday:

Breakfast: sugar free yogurt with peanut butter, cocoa powder and stevia
Lunch: beef fried in ghee with vegetables.
Dinner: a hamburger with bacon, egg and cheese.

Saturday:

Breakfast: ham and cheese omelet with vegetables.
Lunch: sliced ham and cheese with nuts.
Dinner: white fish, eggs and spinach cooked in vegetable oil.

Sunday

Breakfast: fried eggs with bacon and mushrooms
Lunch: burger with salsa, cheese and guacamole.
Dinner: steak and eggs with a side dish.

30 DAYS WEIGHT- LOSS CHALLENGE

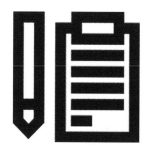

LOSE WEIGHT WITH EASY AND DELICIOUS KETO RECIPES

If we are talking about food that will bring your body and brain the most benefits, then first of all, we mention healthy dishes prepared with love, and cooked from exclusively high quality and healthy ingredients. If you are used to eating in cafes and restaurants, try an experiment: start cooking by yourself, and after 3 months, check the difference in your body, general health condition and feelings.

The modern pace of life does not leave us even an hour a day to cook homemade meals and we always call at the supermarket and buy convenience food. It is always fast, tasty and you there is no need in making extra effort to cook. But food from the supermarket contains a lot of additives, preservatives, colorings and as a result you gain extra weight and health problems. Now it is high time to break this habit to buy everything from the supermarket. Let's cook healthy and nutritious homemade meals.

Everybody agrees that the most wholesome food is cooked at home, for one simple reason - we know what ingredients and how much we use when cooking.

In our special chapter we prepared for you 40 healthy, easy and delicious keto-friendly recipes that will help you to lose extra weight and boost your health. All meals are packed with all necessary useful substances and minerals. The recipes are followed by step-by-step instructions, detailed calorie content and recommendations.

Keep a balanced diet, do physical exercises, cook wholesome meals and be healthy!

BREAKFAST

Coconut porridge

Preparation time: 15 minutes

Servings – 4

Kcal: 487

Carbs: 4g l 0.14oz. l Fats: 49g l 1.72oz. l Proteins: 9g l 0.31oz.

Ingredients:

- 4 eggs (beaten)
- 4 tbsp. / 100g coconut Flour
- 1ts. / 8 g Psyllium
- Salt
- ½ cup / 120 g butter / coconut oil
- 1 ½ cup / 225g coconut cream

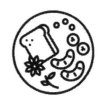

Preparation steps:

1. Combine the eggs, coconut flour, psyllium and salt in a small bowl.

2. Melt the butter and coconut cream over low heat and then slowly pour them into the egg mixture, stirring continuously. Beat the mixture to a thick consistency of sour cream.

3. Serve the dish with coconut milk or cream. Add some fresh or frozen berries to the porridge.

Enjoy your meal!

Omelet with Cheddar cheese

Preparation time: 15 minutes

Servings – 2

Kcal: 897

Carbs: 4g l 0.14 oz. l Fats: 80g l 2.82 oz. l Proteins: 40g l 1.41 oz.

Ingredients:

- 75 g / 5tbsp. butter
- 6 eggs
- 2 cups / 200 g Cheddar Cheese
- Salt and pepper
- chopped or grated cheddar cheese

Preparation steps:

1. Beat the eggs until smooth consistency.

2. Add half a serving of crushed Cheddar cheese. Sprinkle with salt and pepper to taste.

3. Melt the butter in a hot skillet and pour the egg mixture into it.

4. Wait a few minutes until the omelet thickens.

5. Reduce heat and continue to fry omelet until it is almost ready.

6. Add the rest of the chopped cheese. Then fold the omelet in half and immediately serve

Flax pancakes

Preparation time: 20 minutes

Servings – 3

Kcal: 303

Carbs: 1g l 0.03 oz. l Fats: 8g l 0.28 oz. l Proteins: 2g l 0.07 oz.

Ingredients:

- 2/3 cup / 150 g fat sour cream

- 4 eggs

- ½ tsp. / 4g salt

- 1 tsp. / 6g baking powder

- 2,5tbsp. / 50 g room temperature butter

- 6 tsp. / 65g ground flax seeds

- sweetener to taste

- 20 g / 2tbsp. coconut oil

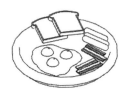

Preparation steps:

1. Using a mixer, beat the butter, add the eggs, sour cream, baking powder, salt and sweetener and beat until smooth all together.

2. Add one spoonful of flax seeds and keep whisking.

3. The dough should turn out as it is for pancakes, that is, as thick sour cream.

4. Heat the pan, put the oil and fry as usual. But lay out the circles thickly and about 4 cm in diameter, because they are spreading out and getting bigger.

5. Fry over low heat, otherwise burn.

6. Serve with whipped cream.

Leftover Egg Muffins

Preparation time: 30 minutes
Servings – 12
Kcal: 106
Carbs: 2g l oz. l Fats: 6g l oz. l Proteins: 11g l oz.

Ingredients:

- ½ cup / 100 g grated cheese
- 12 whites of large eggs (CO)
- 2 small peppers, cut into squares
- 6 feathers of green onions
- salt, pepper, other spices to taste

Preparation steps:

1. Preheat the oven to 180 °C / 356 °F.
2. Mix psyllium with a sweetener.
3. Drizzle the muffin mold with cooking spray or oil.
4. Put peppers and onions inside each pan.
5. Beat the whites and a half of grated cheese, with a fork or whisk, add salt and pepper to taste.
6. Pour the mixture into 12 molds and sprinkle with the remaining cheese and bake for 20 minutes.
7. Serve with chopped parsley.

Cheese rolls with cauliflower

Preparation time: 30 minutes

Servings – 3

Kcal: 190

Carbs: 3g l 0.10oz. l Fats: 14g l 0.49oz. l Proteins: 13g l 0.45oz.

Ingredients:

- 3.5oz. / 90 g cauliflower (can be frozen)

- 4 eggs, separated proteins and yolks

- 1 clove of garlic, crushed

- 2 pieces of processed cheese, grated

- ¼ cup / 50 g cheese, grated

- 2,5 tbsp. / 50g homemade mayonnaise

- salt to taste

- black pepper to taste

- 1 bunch of greens, chop finely

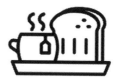

Preparation steps:

1. Blanch cauliflower for 5 minutes, then chop it in a food processor.

2. Preheat the oven to 180°C / 356 °F.

3. Beat the whites to a lush foam and set aside.

4. Mix the cabbage with the yolks, and then carefully mix the whipped whites into them.

5. Cover the baking sheet with a teflon rug or parchment paper.

6. Place the mixture all over the baking sheet and level it with a spatula.

7. Transfer it in the oven for 15 minutes.

8. For the filling: mix all the grated cheese with garlic, spices, salt, herbs and homemade mayonnaise.

9. Carefully shift the base for the roll onto the cling film

10. Put the filling on the base and level it with a spatula.

11. Carefully wrap the roll.

12. Cut the roll into portions and lay on a plate.

Omelet with bacon and avocado

Preparation time: 10 minutes

Servings – 3

Kcal: 125

Carbs: 3g l 0.10oz. l Fats: 9g l 0.31oz. l Proteins: 7g l 0.24oz.

Ingredients:

- 6 eggs
- 1 cup / 200 g sausages, chopped
- ½ cup / 100 g milk
- 1 onion, chop
- 2 tomatoes, chop
- salt and pepper to taste
- 6 strips of bacon
- 1 avocado

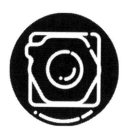

Preparation steps:

1. Fry the strips of bacon and set them aside.
2. In the same pan, slightly fry the onion and sausage. Add tomatoes
3. Beat the eggs and milk with a fork.
4. Add salt and pepper and pour gently into the pan.
5. After 1-2 minutes, reduce the heat and cover the omelet with a lid.
6. Cook it for 10 minutes
7. Place scrambled eggs, fried bacon and avocado slices on serving plates.

Cream pancakes

Preparation time: 20 minutes
Servings – 8
Kcal: 303
Carbs: 7g l 0.24oz. l Fats: 29g l 1.02oz. l Proteins: 9g l 0.31oz.

Ingredients:

- 1 cup / 225g cream cheese
- 3 tbsp. / 60g almond flour
- 4 tbsp. / 57g butter, melt
- 6 eggs separate the whites from the yolks
- 1 tsp. / 8g sweetener (or to taste)
- 1 tsp. / 6ml vanilla extract

Preparation steps:

1. Combine the yolks, melted butter, cream cheese, sweetener and vanilla extract with a mixer to combine all the ingredients.

2. Add flour to the mixture and stir thoroughly.

3. In a separate bowl, beat the whites until fluffy foam, about 5-7 minutes.

4. Add a third of the whites to the dough and gently mix them. Then add the second third of the whites, mix and add the rest to the dough. Mix everything carefully.

5. Sprinkle the pan with any oil.

6. Spread the dough in the pan when it is warm enough. Then reduce heat to medium. Pancakes will not tend to spread, so they need some help to make them not too lush.

7. As soon as the entire surface of the pancake is covered with bubbles, you can gently turn the pancake over. The dough is more tender than usual, so proceed gently.

8. Bake for about a couple of minutes.

Frittata with pink salmon and broccoli

Preparation time: 15 minutes

Servings – 3

Kcal: 134

Carbs: 4g l 0.14 oz. l Fats: 8g l 0.28 oz. l Proteins: 13g l 0.45 oz.

Ingredients:

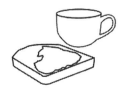

- 6 eggs
- 25 g / 1tbsp. butter
- 1 1/5 cup / 200 g broccoli
- 1 can / 280g of pink salmon cut into pieces
- 1/32 cup / 100 ml whole milk
- 1 tbsp. / 7g herbs,
- 2 green onion feathers, chopped
- black pepper to taste
- ½ cup / 60 g hard cheese, grate

Preparation steps:

1. Blanch broccoli in boiling salted water for 4 minutes. Place in a colander and let drain.

2. Beat eggs and milk slightly, add onion and black pepper to the mixture.

3. Heat butter in a frying pan with a heat-resistant handle and pour the egg mixture into it.

4. Put the pieces of fish and broccoli on top, slightly sinking in the mixture

5. Preheat oven to 190 °C / 374 °F. Cook for 4-5 minutes until the top of the frittata is almost frozen.

6. Sprinkle the dish with grated cheese and put in the oven for 2-3 minutes, until the top turns golden.

7. Sprinkle with herbs

8. Serve with tomatoes.

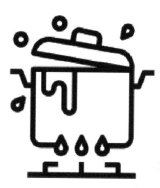

Milk free latte

Preparation time: 5 minutes

Servings – 2

Kcal: 192

Carbs: 1g l 0.03 oz. l Fats: 18g l 0.63 oz. l Proteins: 6g l 0.21 oz.

Ingredients:

- 2 eggs
- 2 tbsp. / 35g Coconut oil
- 1 ½ cup / 350 ml boiling water
- Vanilla extract
- 1 tsp. / 5g Ginger

Preparation steps:

1. Mix the latte ingredients in a blender.
2. Act fast so the eggs don't manage to boil in boiling water that you have added to it!
3. Drink a latte immediately after cooking enjoying its incredible taste.

Homemade burgers

Preparation time: 30 minutes

Servings – 3

Kcal: 255

Carbs: 4g l 0.14 oz. l Fats: 21g l 0.74 oz. l Proteins: 15g l 0.52 oz.

Ingredients:

For pancakes:

- 6 eggs
- 3 tbsp. /75g peanut flour
- 50 grams / 2tbsp. of butter, melted
- salt, black pepper to taste

For filling:

- 9 bacon strips
- 3 eggs

Preparation steps:

1. Mix the ingredients for the pancakes and cook as usual. It is better to use silicone molds for pancakes or scrambled eggs to make them perfectly round.

2. Fry three eggs. It is also advisable to use forms.

3. Roast bacon.

4. Combine all the ingredients in the form of a burger, use additionally everything you want: herbs, cucumbers, cheese or salsa sauce.

LUNCH

Meat casserole

Preparation time: 45 minutes

Servings – 6

Kcal: 942

Carbs: 7g l 0.24 oz. l Fats: 82g l 2.89 oz. l Proteins: 45g l 1.58 oz.

Ingredients:

- 1 1/3 cup / 300 g bacon
- 24 oz. / 675g ground beef
- 3 pickled cucumbers, finely chopped
- 2 tomatoes, diced
- 2 chopped garlic clove (optional)
- Salt and pepper
- 3 cups / 300 g Cheddar Cheese, grated
- 3 eggs
- 1 ½ cup / 335 ml fat Cream
- 3 tbsp. / 60 ml Tomato sauce

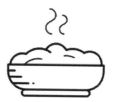

Preparation steps:

1. Preheat the oven to 200 ° C. / 392 °F. Grease the casserole mold with oil or cooking spray.

2. Fry the bacon in a large skillet until crispy. Lay out the bacon on a separate plate.

3. Increase the temperature slightly and using the same frying pan fry the ground beef until cooked through.

4. Add pickled cucumbers, tomatoes, chopped garlic, salt, pepper and 2/3 of cheese.

5. Place fried mince and bacon in a mold for casserole.

6. In a big bowl mix eggs, cream and tomato sauce. Add herbs and spices to taste.

7. Pour the egg mixture into the baking dish.

8. Sprinkle with the remaining cheese.

9. Bake in the oven for approximately 20-25 minutes to a delicious golden-brown crust.

10. Serve with lettuce and olive oil.

Chicken with Tonnato sauce

Preparation time: 35 minutes

Servings – 4

Kcal: 667

Carbs: 2g l 0.07oz. l Fats: 54g l 1.90 oz. l Proteins: 46g l 1.62 oz.

Ingredients:

For the Tonnato sauce

- 2 tbsp. / 20g Capers
- 4 oz. / 110 g canned tuna in olive oil
- 2 cups / 60 g Basil finely chopped
- 1 tsp. / 9g dried parsley
- 2 garlic cloves
- 2 tbsp. / 24 ml Lemon juice
- ½ cup / 125 ml mayonnaise
- 4 tbsp. / 60 ml olive oil
- Salt
- Ground black pepper

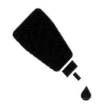

For chicken

- 25 oz. / 700g chicken breast
- Water
- Salt
- 7oz. / 200g greenery

Preparation steps:

1. Using a hand blender combine all the ingredients for the sauce.

2. Put the chicken breasts in a pan with slightly salted water. (If you use

3. cooked chicken, then skip this step.) Bring water to a boil and remove foam formed on the surface.

4. Cook the chicken over medium heat for 15 minutes until is done.

5. Give chicken breasts before slicing to "rest" for at least 10 minutes.

6. Put leafy greens on a plate, place sliced chicken above. Pour over the sauce.

7. Serve with capers and a slice of fresh lemon.

Pork skewers with mashed potatoes and green sauce

Preparation time: 30 minutes

Servings – 4

Kcal: 980

Carbs: 7g l 0.24 oz. l Fats: 93g l 3.28 oz. l Proteins: 30g l 1.05 oz.

Ingredients:

Pork skewers

- 🍽 16 oz. / 450 g pork shoulder
- 🍽 1tbsp. / 15g Ranch Sauce
- 🍽 1 tsp. / 4g Sea salt
- 🍽 1 tbsp. / 15 ml olive oil

Cauliflower puree

- 🍽 23oz. / 650 g Cauliflower
- 🍽 2/3 cup / 150 g butter
- 🍽 ½ cup / 60 g Parmesan, grated
- 🍽 Salt and pepper

Green sauce

- 🍽 4 cups / 100 g Parsley, finely chopped fresh parsley
- 🍽 23 tbsp. / 50 g cilantro, finely chopped fresh cilantro or basil
- 🍽 ½ lemon juice

- 🍽 2 tbsp. / 50g capers
- 🍽 2 garlic cloves
- 🍽 2/3 cup / 150 ml olive oil
- 🍽 1 tsp. / 4g Sea salt
- 🍽 Ground black pepper

Preparation steps:

1. Put all the ingredients in the bowl and mix using a hand blender.

2. Cut the pork shoulder along into slices about 2.5 cm thick. Season with ranch sauce. String meat on wooden skewers such a length that the resulting kebabs fit in a pan.

3. Heat the frying pan, add olive oil and fry kebabs for several minutes on each side until complete readiness.

4. Divide cauliflower into buds. Peel, remove the stem and cut into small pieces.

5. Place the cauliflower for a couple of minutes in boiling slightly salted water until inflorescences become softer, but not losing their shape.

6. Drain the water. To make mashed potatoes denser, put the cauliflower on a clean towel and squeeze the excess fluid thoroughly.

7. Put the cauliflower in a mixer or food processor and combine with butter and parmesan.

8. Season with salt and pepper to taste.

Fried pork with green pepper

Preparation time: 20 minutes

Servings – 2

Kcal: 838

Carbs: 5g l 0.17 oz. l Fats: 78g l 2.75oz. l Proteins: 29g l 1.02 oz.

Ingredients:

- 🍽 10.5 oz. / 300 g pork shoulder
- 🍽 2 green bell pepper
- 🍽 2 green onions
- 🍽 ½ cup / 110 g butter
- 🍽 2 tbsp. / 30g almonds
- 🍽 1 tsp. / 12g Chili pasta
- 🍽 Salt and pepper

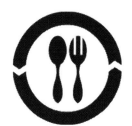

Preparation steps:

1. Cut the pork into thin strips.

2. Chop pepper and chives. Melt the butter in a frying pan. Leave some part of butter for serving.

3. Sauté the pork strips over high heat for a few minutes. Add vegetables and chili paste. Continue frying, stirring for some a couple of minutes. Season with salt and pepper.

4. Serve with almond and butter.

Salmon with spinach

Preparation time: 15 minutes

Servings – 2

Kcal: 780

Carbs: 2g l 0.07oz. l Fats: 70g l 2.46 oz. l Proteins: 37g l 1.31 oz.

Ingredients:

- 27,5oz. / 350g Salmon, sliced

- 2 tbsp. / 50g Butter (for frying)

- 3 tbsp. / 70 g butter

- 1 Red bell pepper

- 2 cups / 70 g Spinach (young)

- Salt and pepper

Preparation steps:

1. Put the pan over medium heat, add the butter. Add salmon slices and fry for several minutes on each side.

2. When the salmon is almost ready, reduce the fire. Add salt and pepper to your taste.

3. Place cooked salmon slices on top and garnish them with softened creamy butter, bell pepper, and spinach, and serve.

Tomato soup

Preparation time: 1 hour 30 minutes

Servings – 6

Kcal: 404

Carbs: 4 g l 0.14 oz. l Fats: 35g l 1.23 oz. l Proteins: 20g l 0.71oz.

Ingredients:

- 28,2 oz. / 800 g chicken wings
- 9 cups / 1½ liters of water
- 1 small onion
- 4 leek leaves
- 3/8 cup / 40 g celery
- 1 cup / 200 ml cream, 36%
- 1 carrot
- 2 bay leaves
- ½ cup / 100 ml olive oil
- 1 parsley root
- 1 head garlic
- 3 tbsp. / 45ml of tomato puree
- Parsley leaves
- salt, black pepper, paprika to taste
- Fresh basil

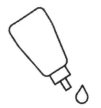

Preparation steps:

1. Rinse the chicken wings and vegetables. Throw it in salted boiling water and bring to boil.

2. After, add the chopped bay leaves, leek leaves, onion to the pan. Add seasonings and simmer for one hour.

3. Strain the keto soup. Pour the broth back into the pan and set aside the rest. Add tomato puree, olive oil and cream to the pan. Bring back over medium heat again.

4. Separate the wings from the bones and add to the soup pot.

5. Slice boiled carrots, celery and parsley root and add to the soup. Add herbs and spices. Cut the leaves of parsley and basil and put them in the soup.

6. Cook for 5 minutes.

7. Pour into plates and sprinkle with chopped parsley.

Orange baked cauliflower soup

Preparation time: 30 minutes

Servings – 4

Kcal: 496

Carbs: 9g l 0.31oz. l Fats: 42g l 1.48 oz. l Proteins: 6g l 0.21 oz.

Ingredients:

- 1 kg / 2lb cauliflower
- 2 heads of garlic
- 1 small red onion
- 1 tsp. / 7g caraway seeds (need to be fried and chopped)
- 2 tsp. / 12g turmeric
- 1 tsp. / 6g curry powder
- 1 tsp. / 6g ground bell pepper
- fresh coriander, bunch
- 1 can / 250 ml coconut milk
- 2 cups / 500 ml of meat broth
- salt and black pepper to taste
- 4 tbsp. / 60 ml olive oil
- 10 mint leaves for sprinkling, optional
- 1 tbsp. / 15ml of coconut oil for frying

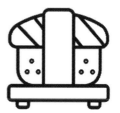

Preparation steps:

1. Separate the stems of cauliflower from inflorescences. Season with salt and pepper.

2. Bake cauliflower in an oven preheated to 200°C /392 °F for 25 minutes.

3. Remove the baked cauliflower from the oven and chop finely.

4. Cut coriander and onions, fry them in coconut oil. Then add spices, chopped cauliflower and fry for a couple of minutes.

5. Transfer vegetables to the pan, pour the broth, coconut milk and cook for 10 minutes. Salt and pepper, if necessary.

6. Keto soup is ready. If desired, sprinkle with mint leaves before serving.

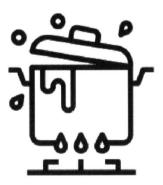

Green asparagus soup with green peas and dill

Preparation time: 30 minutes

Servings – 1

Kcal: 319

Carbs: 10g l 0.35oz. l Fats: 27g l 0.95oz. l Proteins: 9g l 0.31oz.

Ingredients:

- 🍽 2 cups / 500 ml chicken stock
- 🍽 1,5 tbsp. / 30 g butter
- 🍽 17.6 oz. / 500 g green asparagus
- 🍽 ¼ cup / 30 g onions
- 🍽 1 cup / 210 ml cream 36%
- 🍽 1 garlic clove
- 🍽 8.8. oz / 250 g green peas, fresh or frozen
- 🍽 20 mint leaves
- 🍽 salt and pepper to taste
- 🍽 dill, bunch

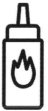

Preparation steps:

1. Dice onion and garlic and fry in butter.

2. Transfer the onions and garlic into the pan, pour the meat broth, add asparagus and cook for 20 minutes.

3. Strain the broth to separate the vegetables.

4. Mix vegetables and rub them through a sieve.

5. Boil peas in strained broth (about 3 minutes).

6. Add grated vegetables, mint, half diced dill to the broth and peas. Salt, pepper and mix well.

7. Bring the soup to a boil.

8. Serve keto soup with sprinkled dill and chili.

Pork chops with vegetables

Preparation time: 40 minutes

Servings – 3

Kcal: 439

Carbs: 2g l 0.07oz. l Fats: 24g l 0.84 oz. l Proteins: 50g l 1.76 oz.

Ingredients:

- 17.6 oz. / 500g Pork chops
- ¼ cup / 60g Flax Seeds
- 3 tbsp. / Coconut Oil
- 2tsp. / 16g Caraway seeds
- 1tsp. / 6g Coriander
- 1 tsp. / 6g Cardamom
- Salt and pepper
- 1 Sweet pepper
- 1 Onion
- 2 Celery Stalks
- ¼ cup / 65 ml White wine

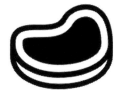

Preparation steps:

1. Rub the pork chops with salt and pepper.

2. In a wide bowl, combine flax, coriander, cardamom and caraway seeds and then roll each piece of meat in spices on both sides.

3. Melt coconut oil in a pan. When the it melts and begins to evaporate, put the pork chops in the pan. Fry the meat until the crust becomes crispy and golden.

4. Place the finished pork chops onto the foil. The meat should "rest"

5. Put chopped vegetables in the oil and meat juice. Season them with salt and pepper. When frying vegetables, add white wine.

6. Serve with chopped greenery.

Salmon kish with spinach

Preparation time: 30 minutes

Servings – 4

Kcal:

Carbs: 3g l 0.10 oz. l Fats: 42g l 1.48 oz. l Proteins: 29g l 1.01 oz.

Ingredients:

For crust:

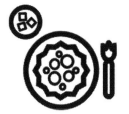

- 20g / 1 tbsp. Psyllium
- 1 egg
- ½ tbsp. / 4g Soda
- 4 tbsp. / 90g Butter
- 90g / 3,5 tbsp. Coconut Flour

For filling:

- 10g Dill
- 2 eggs
- 3.8 oz. / 110g Salmon, raw
- ½ cup / 150 ml Cream 33%
- Salt, pepper - to taste.

Preparation steps:

1. Combine psyllium, egg, soda, butter, coconut flour.

2. Put the dough into the mold, form a base with sides approximately 2 cm.

3. Place in a preheated oven to 180°C / 356 °F for 10 min.

4. Remove from the oven, add the diced salmon.

5. In a bowl, combine eggs, cream, salt, pepper, chopped dill. Mix well.

6. Fill the salmon just below the height of the sides of the dough.

7. Bake at 170 ° C / 338 °F for 30-35 minutes or until golden brown.

DINNER

Salmon with mushrooms in cream cheese sauce

Preparation time: 30 minutes
Servings – 3
Kcal: 162
Carbs: 4g l 0.14oz. l Fats: 10g l 0.35oz. l Proteins: 14g l 0.49 oz.

Ingredients:

- 17.6oz. / 500g salmon
- ½ cup / 100g leek
- ½ cup / 150 ml cream
- Sea salt
- Parsley
- 2,5 tbsp. / 40 ml olive oil
- 2 2/3 cup / 200g champignons
- 1 cup / 120 processed cheese
- 2 garlic cloves

Preparation steps:

1. Wash the salmon fillet and cut into small pieces, about 4x4 centimeters. Pour olive (sunflower) oil into the pan and put the fish.

2. Fry slices of salmon in oil on all sides for 10 minutes.

3. Cut the leek into thin rings.

4. Peel the mushrooms and cut into pieces.

5. Transfer the fried salmon from the pan to the plate. Pour olive oil in the frying pan and put the chopped leeks and mushrooms. Fry for 5-7 minutes.

6. Add cream and processed cheese to leek and mushrooms.

7. Stir the mushrooms, leeks, cream and cream cheese. You can add dry white wine, it will turn out even tastier.

8. Add salt to taste and season with spices if necessary.

9. In the creamy cheese sauce, put the pieces of fried salmon and simmer in a pan for five minutes.

10. Serve with any side dish.

Salmon and spinach pie

Preparation time: 45 minutes

Servings – 5

Kcal: 322

Carbs: 4g l 0.14oz. l Fats: 25g l 0.88 oz. l Proteins: 17g l 0.59 oz.

Ingredients:

- 1 ½ cup / 192g almond flour
- ¼ cup / 72g Sesame seeds
- 1 tbsp. / 25g Psyllium (flour)
- ½ cup / 100g Butter
- 5 eggs
- 1 1/3 cup / 300g frozen Spinach
- 2 cups / 200g Grated cheese
- 1 cup / 200g Fat sour cream
- 7 oz. / 200g Cold smoked salmon, thinly chopped
- 5.2 oz. / 150g/ shrimps
- ½ cup / 100g Mayonnaise
- Dill, 1 bunch
- Salt
- Pepper, seasoning to taste

Preparation steps:

1. Thaw out spinach. Preheat the oven to 200 °C / 392 °F

2. Cook the dough. Mix almond flour, psyllium and sesame seeds. Heat the oil (in a water bath, or in the microwave) to a semi-liquid state. It should not be hot. Mix the butter with one egg well, pour it all into the flour and knead the dough thoroughly. It should turn out very dense, almost like clay.

3. Take a cake pan with removable edges, put baking paper on the bottom, grease the sides with oil and put the dough there. The dough is very dense, so some physical effort will be required. As a result, you should get a very thin bottom and bumpers 1.5-2 cm high. Put the mold in the oven for 8 minutes.

4. Cook the filling: squeeze out excess water from the thawed spinach, add the remaining 4 eggs, sour cream and grated cheese. Mix thoroughly, season with salt, pepper, and seasonings.

5. Take out the form with the dough from the oven, let it cool slightly and pour half of the resulting filling into it. Gently spread the salmon slices on top and pour the second half of the filling on them.

6. Put in the oven for 25-30 minutes.

7. Garnish the pie with shrimps add the mayonnaise on top and sprinkle with chopped dill.

Bacon and cheese balls

Preparation time: 20 minutes

Servings – 8

Kcal: 283

Carbs: 2g l 0.07oz. l Fats: 27g l 0.95 oz. l Proteins: 8g l 0.28 oz.

Ingredients:

- 🍽 5.2oz. / 150 g Bacon
- 🍽 1 tbsp. / 20g Butter
- 🍽 2/3 cup / 150 g Cream Cheese
- 🍽 1 ½ cup / 150 g Cheddar Cheese
- 🍽 50 g / 2tbsp. butter, room temperature
- 🍽 Pepper
- 🍽 Chili flakes

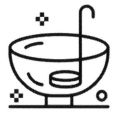

Preparation steps:

1. Fry the bacon in butter until rosy crusts. Transfer it from the frying pan to a paper towel and let cool completely.

2. Break or chop the cooled bacon into small pieces and place in a bowl of medium size.

3. In a large bowl, mix leftover bacon grease and the rest of the ingredients with the help of a food processor.

4. Place a large bowl in the refrigerator for 15 minutes.

5. Use 2 spoons to make 24 balls the size of a walnut. Roll in chopped bacon and serve.

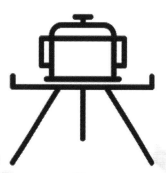

Bacon and zucchini pancakes

Preparation time: 25 minutes

Servings – 2

Kcal: 455

Carbs: 5g l 0.17 oz. l Fats: 39g l 1.37 oz. l Proteins: 18g l 0.63 oz.

Ingredients:

- 14 oz. / 400 g Zucchini
- 2 eggs
- ¼ cup / 60 g Bacon (sugar free)
- 2 tbsp. / 55g Flax flour
- 2 Tbsp. / 30ml Olive Oil (Extra Virgin

Preparation steps:

1. Cook the zucchini - grate, put in a colander and sprinkle with salt. Leave the colander for 20 minutes over the sink or pan, then squeeze the moisture out.

2. Over medium heat, heat the oil, spread the pieces of bacon and fry for several minutes.

3. In the container, mix the bacon, zucchini, egg and flour.

4. Fry the pancakes in the same pan for several minutes on each side.

Avocado with fish

Preparation time: 5 minutes
Servings – 2
Kcal: 422
Carbs: 13g l 0.45 oz. l Fats: 30g l 1.05 oz. l Proteins: 9g l 0.31oz.

Ingredients:

- 🍽 2 avocadoes
- 🍽 7oz. / 200g salmon
- 🍽 ½ cup / 70g onion
- 🍽 2 tbsp. / 40g keto mayonnaise

Preparation steps:

1. Cut the avocado, remove the bone. Scoop out the pulp with a spoon, leaving half a centimeter on the rind.

2. Mash the trout flesh with a fork (it can be fresh, smoked or canned).

3. Combine fish with finely chopped onions, salt and pepper to taste, add keto mayonnaise.

4. Stuff the avocado halves with obtained mixture.

P.S. A simplified version - select the whole pulp with a spoon and just make the salad in a separate container.

Zucchini casserole with mince

Preparation time: 45 minutes

Servings – 4

Kcal:

Carbs: 10g l 0.35 oz. l Fats: 47g l 1.65oz. l Proteins: 30g l 1.05 oz.

Ingredients:

- 🍽 14oz. / 400 g ground meat (pork + beef)
- 🍽 1 big zucchini
- 🍽 2/3 cup / 160 ml Sour Cream
- 🍽 2/3 cup / 80 g Cheese
- 🍽 1 egg
- 🍽 Greens (parsley and dill)

Preparation steps:

1. Rub the zucchini on a coarse grater, salt, put on a sieve, after 10 minutes squeeze out excess water.

2. In the container, mix the stuffing, zucchini, cheese, egg and greens.

3. Put the mass in a baking dish, put it in preheated up to 180 °C / 356 °F oven for 30 minutes.

4. At the very end, you can turn on convection for a few minutes for the crust on top.

Goulash

Preparation time: 50 minutes

Servings – 4

Kcal: 462

Carbs: 14g l 0.49oz. l Fats: 34g l 2.61oz. l Proteins: 27g l 0.95 oz.

Ingredients:

- 14.1. oz / 400 g Beef (minced meat)
- 21.1oz. / 600 zucchinis
- 1 tbsp. / 15 ml Olive Oil
- 2 Onions
- 4 garlic cloves
- 2-3 tbsp. / 45g sugar-free tomato paste / (1 tomato mashed)
- 1 red bell pepper
- 1 cup / 250 ml beef broth
- green basil
- salt, pepper

Preparation steps:

1. Add ground beef, onions and garlic to the saucepan and sauté over medium heat, stirring the minced meat.

2. After the meat changes color, add the remaining ingredients to the pan and bring to a boil.

3. Reduce to a boil, cover and cook for 20 minutes, stirring occasionally, or until zucchini reaches desired degree of softness.

Hawaiian gluten free pizza

Preparation time: 45 minutes

Servings – 6

Kcal: 193

Carbs: 10g l 0.35 oz. l Fats: 15g l 0.52 oz. l Proteins: 23g l 0.81 oz.

Ingredients:

For base:

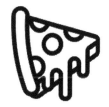

- 12 heads of cauliflower
- 1 egg
- 1 cup / 100 g Mozzarella
- 1 tsp. / 6g Oregano
- 1 garlic clove
- Salt, pepper to taste

For filling:

- ½ cup / 120 ml marinara sauce
- 1 cup / 100 g Mozzarella
- Bacon 3 strips
- pineapple (rings), fresh, (2 pineapples)

Preparation steps:

1. Preheat the oven to 200 °C / 392 °F. Line the baking sheet with parchment paper. Grease it with a thin layer of butter or oil.

2. Divide the cauliflower into inflorescences, then ground it in a blender or a food processor to the state of small grains. Put the cauliflower in the microwave container, cook in the microwave at a maximum power for 4 minutes.

3. Let cool. Squeeze extra water with the help of cheesecloth or sieve.

4. Beat the egg, add spices, grated mozzarella, salt, pepper, mix well.

5. Spread the obtained mass onto a baking tray, form a base for pizza about 1 cm thick. Bake for 20 minutes, take out from the oven.

6. Cook until thickened for 3-4 minutes, turn off, let cool. After that, grind everything with a submersible blender right in the pan - the sauce is ready.

7. Lubricate the base with the sauce, place the toppings, cover with cheese, bake for another 15 minutes.

P.S. you can cook the sauce by yourself. Heat a skillet and add 1 tablespoon of olive oil, add 1-2 garlic cloves, as soon as the garlic begins to blacken - remove it from the pan, add a can of tomatoes in your own juice (no sugar!). Bring the mixture to a boil, add salt, pepper, oregano to taste, you can mix Italian herbs and very preferably fresh basil.

Tuna salad

Preparation time: 12 minutes

Servings – 1

Kcal: 464

Carbs: 14g l 0.49oz. l Fats: 31 l 1.09oz. l Proteins: 4g l 0.14oz.

Ingredients:

Dressing:

- 1 tbsp. / 15 ml olive oil
- 12 tbsp. / 120ml apple vinegar
- Salt, pepper

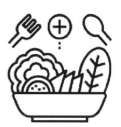

Salad:

- 4 lettuce leaves, big
- 1 tomato
- 1 cucumber
- Avocado

Tuna:

- 1 canned tuna in oil
- 1 tbsp. / 20g natural yogurt
- 1 tbsp. / 20g pesto sauce
- 2 tsp. / 20 ml lemon juice
- Salt, pepper

Preparation steps:

1. Combine vinegar, salt, oil, and pepper.

2. Mix tuna, yogurt, pesto, lemon juice and salt.

3. Put the tuna mixture on the salad, add dressing.

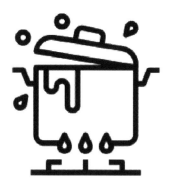

Quesadilla

Preparation time: 15 minutes

Servings – 2

Kcal: 505

Carbs: 4g l 0.14 oz. l Fats: 38g l 1.34oz. l Proteins: 36g l 1.26 oz.

Ingredients:

- 1 cup / 100 g mozzarella
- 1 cup / 100 g Cheddar Cheese
- 5.2oz. / 150 g Ready chicken (boiled or baked)
- 12 Bulgarian Peppers
- 12 Tomato
- 1 tbsp. / 15g Chives

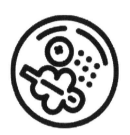

Preparation steps:

1. Preheat the oven to 200 °C / 392 °F. Place the parchment on a baking tray, grease the parchment with a thin layer of oil. Grate cheeses, mix, put on a parchment in the shape of a circle.

2. Bake for 5 minutes

3. Lay out the pieces of chicken on one half of the baked cheese flatbread. Add vegetables.

4. Fold in half and bake for 6-8 minutes.

5. Remove from the oven, let cool, cut into portions.

6. Serve with sour cream, guacamole or salsa.

DESSERTS / SNACKS

Gluten and lactose free cheesecake

Preparation time: 30 minutes

Servings – 16

Kcal: 380

Carbs: 9g l 0.31oz. l Fats: 35g l 1.23 oz. l Proteins: 9g l 0.31 oz.

Ingredients:

Base:

- 7/8 cup / 100g walnuts
- 1 cup / 130g almond flour
- ½ cup / 60g coconut flour
- Sea salt

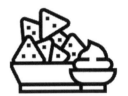

Filling:

- 3 cups / 400g cashew nuts
- ¾ cup / 180 ml coconut milk
- ½ cup / 100g coconut oil
- 1 tbsp. / 15 ml vanilla extract
- 1/3 cup / 35g sugar free cocoa powder
- 3 tbsp. / 45ml lemon juice
- 4 tbsp. / 80g sweetener

Topping:

- 1 cup / 85g black chocolate
- 1/3 cup / 80 ml coconut milk

Preparation steps:

1. Place all the ingredients for the base in a blender (you need a large one with horizontal blades) and grind to a state of a mixture of fine crumbs. Spread everything in 23 cm. Tamp.

2. In the same blender, mix all the ingredients for filling. Pulse until homogeneous mass is formed, approximately 2-5 minutes, sometimes you can use a spatula to collect the mass from the walls.

3. Pour the mixture into a mold in which the base is already set. Leave in the freezer for 2 hours.

4. In a water bath heat coconut milk and chocolate (break into pieces), melt and mix everything. Pour on top of the frozen mass.

5. Send in the freezer for another hour.

Gluten free muffins

Preparation time: 25 minutes

Servings – 12

Kcal: 150

Carbs: 1g l 0.03 oz. l Fats: 12g l 0.42 oz. l Proteins: 10g l 0.35 oz.

Ingredients:

- 5 eggs
- ¾ cup / 160 g cottage cheese, fat
- ¾ cup / 120g ham
- 1 ¼ cup / 120g parmesan
- 2 tbsp. / 50g almond flour
- Salt, pepper to taste

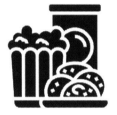

Preparation steps:

1. Preheat the oven to 200 °C / 392 °F.

2. Mix cottage cheese with flour and eggs

3. Dice ham, grate cheese. Mix all the ingredients.

4. Divide the mixture into molds (you need to fill them in about half or a little more)

5. Bake for 20-25 minutes

P.S. There are many options for this dish, the simplest is to remove the cottage cheese, flour and baking powder and instead just add 5 eggs and bake for only 10-12 minutes, you will just get an omelet, but in an interesting and convenient way. You can diversify the filling:

– onion greens

– spinach with cheese

– broccoli with chicken (if meat is left from the broth for example), etc.

Cheese waffles with thyme

Preparation time: 25 minutes

Servings – 4

Kcal: 606

Carbs: 9g l 0.31oz. l Fats: 52g l 1.83 oz. l Proteins: 27g l 0.95 oz.

Ingredients:

- 14oz. / 400 g Cauliflower
- 1 ¼ cup / 280 g cheese
- 4 eggs
- 1 bunch of green onions
- 2 tbsp. / 30 ml Coconut Oil
- 4 tbsp. / 100g Almond flour
- 1 tsp. / 8g Granulated Garlic
- 2 tsp. / 12g Thyme
- Salt and pepper to taste

Preparation steps:

1. Cut cauliflower into inflorescences, finely chop green onions and separate the thyme from the stems. Grind cauliflower in a blender

2. Add green onions and thyme to the mixture. Continue to grind in the "Ripple" mode until everything mixes well. Put the mixture in a large bowl.

3. Add the remaining ingredients, salt and pepper and mix everything thoroughly.

4. Preheat the waffle iron, distribute the mass on the surface of the waffle iron.

5. Cook according to the instructions of the waffle iron.

6. Serve hot.

Homemade chocolate

Preparation time: 15 minutes

Servings – 1

Kcal: 322

Carbs: 4g l 0.14 oz. l Fats: 25g l 0.88 oz. l Proteins: 6g l 0.21 oz.

Ingredients:

- ¾ cup / 180g coconut oil

- ½ cup / 50g cocoa powder

- ¼ cup / 50g cobnuts, fried

- ¼ cup / 50g almonds, fried

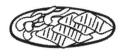

Preparation steps:

1. Melt the butter in a water bath and add cocoa powder.

2. Mix everything until a homogeneous mass is obtained. If you want you can add stevia to taste.

3. Pour some of the chocolate into the silicone mold to just cover the bottom.

4. Then carefully spread the nuts and fill with the remaining chocolate.

5. Cover with cling film or foil and put in the freezer.

Chocolate tart

Preparation time: 25 minutes

Servings – 6

Kcal: 316

Carbs: 13g l 0.45 oz. l Fats: 25g l 0.88 oz. l Proteins: 10g l 0.35 oz.

Ingredients:

- 1 cup / 120g almond flour
- ¾ cup / 80g coconut flour
- 1 egg
- 2 tbsp. / 45g erythritol
- 2 tbsp. / 30g gelatin (powder)
- 1 ¼ cup / 100g dark chocolate(homemade)
- 2 cups / 500 ml fat cream
- 50 ml / 2 tbsp. water
- ¼ cup / 50 g peeled hazelnuts

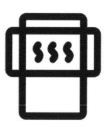

Preparation steps:

1. Mix the egg with coconut and almond flour, knead the dough. Preheat the oven, distribute the dough in a greased form, forming the sides. Bake the workpiece at 180 °C / 356 °F for 20 minutes.

2. Pour gelatin with water, leave to swell.

3. Melt the chocolate in cream, stirring constantly over low heat. Dissolve the gelatin over a small fire, without boiling.

4. Mix chocolate cream, gelatin, sweetener.

5. Pour the mixture into the prepared form, refrigerate for 3 hours.

6. Garnish the frozen tart with hazelnuts, pour chocolate if you wish.

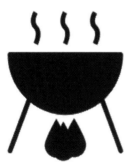

Raspberry lemon ice cream

Preparation time: 20 minutes

Servings – 2

Kcal: 238

Carbs: 2g l 0.07oz. l Fats: 22g l 0.77oz. l Proteins: 5g l 0.17 oz.

Ingredients:

- 3.5oz. / 100 g raspberries;

- ½ lemon juice

- ¼ cup / 58ml coconut oil;

- 250 ml / 1 cup coconut milk;

- ¼ cup / 65ml sour cream;

- ¼ cup / 65ml thick cream;

- 20 drops of liquid stevia.

Preparation steps:

1. Place all the ingredients in a container and liquidize in a blender until raspberries are mixed with other products.

2. Try the mixture to get rid of raspberry seeds. This is important because the seeds in the finished ice cream will irritate the tongue.

3. Pour the mixture into molds and place in the freezer for at least two hours.

4. Serve with melted chocolate and chopped nuts.

Cinnabons

Preparation time: 30 minutes

Servings – 5

Kcal: 308

Carbs: 3g l 0.10 oz. l Fats: 17g l 0.59 oz. l Proteins: 7g l 0.24 oz.

Ingredients:

Dough:

- 🍽 1 cup / 100 g mozzarella cheese;
- 🍽 2/3 cup / 100 g cream cheese;
- 🍽 2 eggs
- 🍽 1 tsp. / 7ml vanillin;
- 🍽 1 tsp. / 6ml liquid stevia;
- 🍽 ¾ cup / 80g coconut flour;
- 🍽 Salt
- 🍽 1 tsp. / 6g baking powder

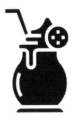

Filling:

- 🍽 ½ cup / 114g butter;
- 🍽 2 tsp. / 15g cinnamon
- 🍽 Stevia to taste

Glazing:

- 🍽 3 tbsp. / 60g fat cream;
- 🍽 2/3 cup / 100g cream cheese;

- 🍽 1 tbsp. / 24g stevia;

- 🍽 vanilla.

Preparation steps:

1. Preheat the oven to 250°C / 482 °Fahrenheit. Mix mozzarella and cream cheese and melt them in the microwave or on the stove over low heat. Stir until smooth consistency. Add the remaining ingredients for the dough to the cheese and mix well.

2. Put the dough on a sheet of parchment paper, cover with another sheet on top and roll it. Slice into strips.

3. Mix melted butter and cinnamon. Spread half the mixture on strips of dough. Roll them and place them on a greased baking sheet. Pour the remaining mixture onto buns on top.

4. Bake for 15-18 minutes.

5. Make icing. Mix the ingredients in a blender. Spread over hot buns.

Pumpkin cookies

Preparation time: 35 minutes
Servings – 4
Kcal: 177
Carbs: 4g l 0.14oz. l Fats: 22g l 0.77oz. l Proteins: 7g l 0.24oz.

Ingredients:

- 3 tbsp. / 60g thick pumpkin puree
- 1 cup / 120g almond flour
- 1 egg
- ¼ cup / 60g melted butter
- 2 tbsp. / 50g stevia to taste
- 1 tbsp./ spice mixes: (cinnamon, nutmeg, cloves, ginger)
- Cinnamon
- 1 tsp. / 5g vanilla extract
- 1/2 tsp. / 3g soda
- 1 tsp. / 6g baking powder
- 2/3 cup / 60g chocolate chips or minced dark chocolate
- 1/3 cup / 40g chopped nuts
- Salt

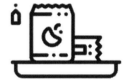

Preparation steps:

1. Mix melted butter (not hot) with pumpkin puree, add an egg, stir thoroughly.

2. Add all spices, salt, stevia, vanilla extract to the liquid mixture, mix well.

3. Add in parts flour with baking powder, soda and mix the dough well. At the end, add chocolate chips and nuts and mix.

4. Spread the dough on a parchment with a measuring spoon, flattening cookies on top. Bake in a preheated oven at 175 °C / 347 °F for 25 min.

Vanilla Frappuccino

Preparation time: 7 minutes
Servings – 1
Kcal: 119
Carbs: 1g l 0.03oz. l Fats: 10g l 0.35oz. l Proteins: 5g l 0.17oz.

Ingredients:

- 1 cup / 200 ml. unsweetened vanilla almond milk;
- 3 tbsp. / 55g fat cream;
- 1 tsp. / 7ml vanilla extract;
- 1 tsp. / 7ml liquid stevia;
- ice;
- whipped cream and chocolate chips for decoration.

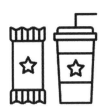

Preparation steps:

1. Beat all ingredients except ice with a blender.
2. Add ice and mix again.
3. Garnish with cream and chocolate chips.

Keto sweet bars

Preparation time: 40 minutes

Servings – 1

Kcal: 226

Carbs: 4g l 0.14 oz. l Fats: 25g l 0.88 oz. l Proteins: 12g l 0.42 oz.

Ingredients:

- 🍽 2/3 cup / 150 g butter
- 🍽 ½ cup / 100 g coconut oil
- 🍽 2 cups / 150 g coconut flakes
- 🍽 3 tbsp. / 45g of peanut paste with a slide
- 🍽 ¾ cup / 100 g chocolate 100%
- 🍽 5-7 tbsp. / 100g erythritol
- 🍽 1 tsp / 8ml vanilla essence

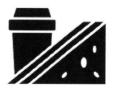

Preparation steps:

1. Melt coconut oil with 2 tablespoons of erythritol, mix thoroughly with coconut flakes. Spread an obtained mass on a baking tray previously lined with parchment paper. Level it up and place in a freezer for 15 minutes.

2. Melt 100g butter with peanut butter and 2 tablespoons of erythritol. Mix thoroughly, and add vanilla extract. Place this mixture over coconut layer and level evenly. Send in a freezer for 20 minutes.

3. Melt chocolate with 3 tablespoons of erythritol and 50g of butter on a water bath or in a microwave. Mix thoroughly. The consistency should be homogeneous and glossy.

4. Get the form with the frozen filling for the bars. Cut the filling into even bars. Prepare a blank sheet of baking paper - put it on the board, which you can then put back into the freezer.

5. With the help of 2 forks dip the bars in chocolate in turns. Place on a clean parchment paper. Transfer the ready bars in a freezer for 1 hour.

Disclaimer

This book contains opinions and ideas of the author and is meant to teach the reader informative and helpful knowledge while due care should be taken by the user in the application of the information provided. The instructions and strategies are possibly not right for every reader and there is no guarantee that they work for everyone. Using this book and implementing the information/recipes therein contained is explicitly your own responsibility and risk. This work with all its contents, does not guarantee correctness, completion, quality or correctness of the provided information. Misinformation or misprints cannot be completely eliminated.

Design: Oliviaprodesign

Picture: Kiian Oksana / www.shutterstock.com